An Essay On Mineral, Animal and Vegetable Poisons ...

Anonymous

Nabu Public Domain Reprints:

You are holding a reproduction of an original work published before 1923 that is in the public domain in the United States of America, and possibly other countries. You may freely copy and distribute this work as no entity (individual or corporate) has a copyright on the body of the work. This book may contain prior copyright references, and library stamps (as most of these works were scanned from library copies). These have been scanned and retained as part of the historical artifact.

This book may have occasional imperfections such as missing or blurred pages, poor pictures, errant marks, etc. that were either part of the original artifact, or were introduced by the scanning process. We believe this work is culturally important, and despite the imperfections, have elected to bring it back into print as part of our continuing commitment to the preservation of printed works worldwide. We appreciate your understanding of the imperfections in the preservation process, and hope you enjoy this valuable book.

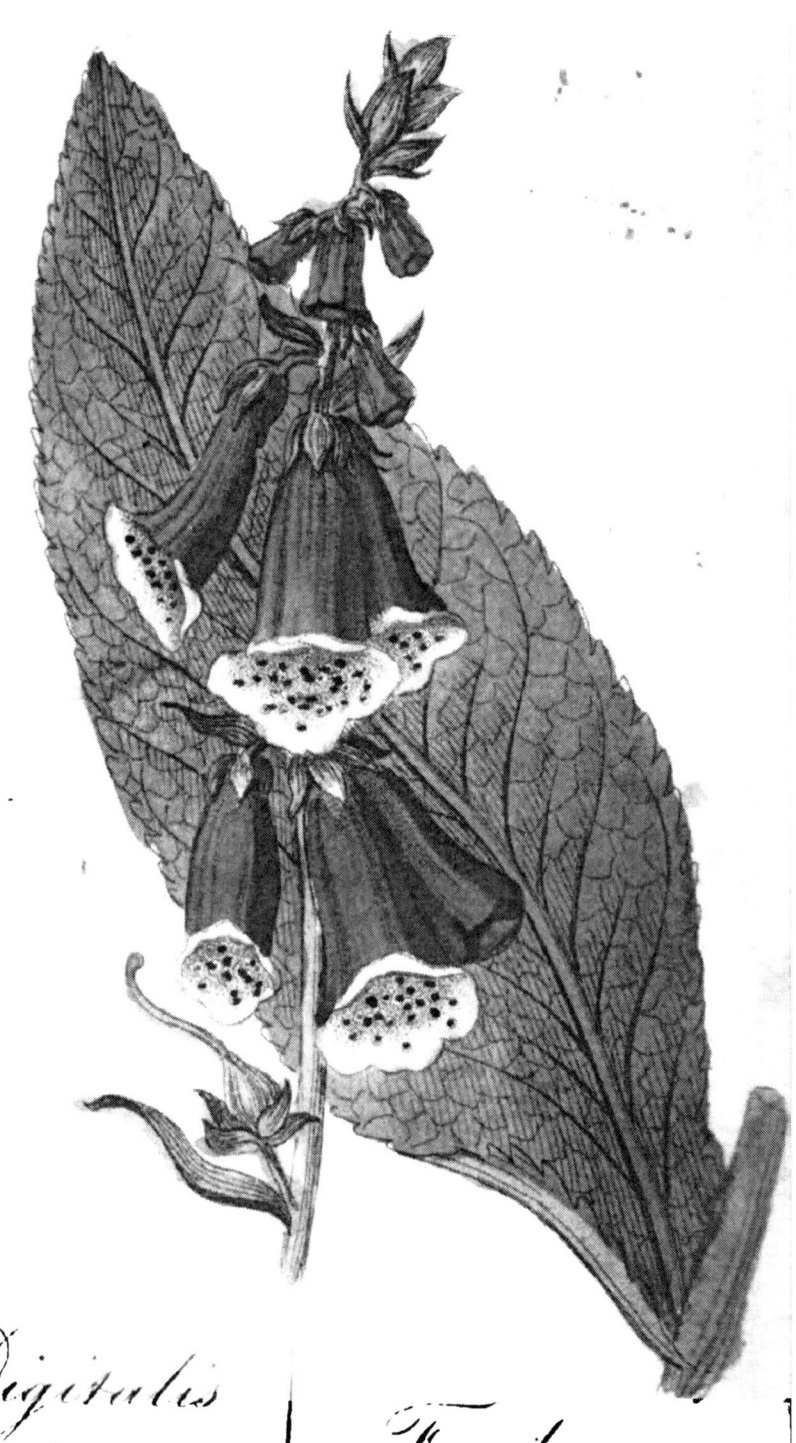

AN ESSAY ON

MINERAL, ANIMAL, AND VEGETABLE POISONS;

IN WHICH
THE SYMPTOMS, MODE OF TREATMENT AND
TESTS OF EACH PARTICULAR POISON,

WITH THE
GENERAL MORBID APPEARANCES on DISSECTION,

ARE CONCISELY DETAILED:

TO WHICH IS ADDED,
AN ACCOUNT OF THE MEANS TO BE EMPLOYED
IN CASES OF SUSPENDED ANIMATION.

Fourth Edition Corrected,
ILLUSTRATED BY THIRTEEN COLOURED PLATES:

PRINTED FOR COX AND SON,
St. Thomas's Street, Southwark;

Sold also by T. and G. Underwood, and Highley, Fleet-Street; Callow and Wilson, Prince's Street, Soho; Simpkin and Marshall, Stationers' Court; Anderson, West Smithfield; John Cox, Berners Street, Oxford Street; W. Stewart, Edinburgh; and J. Cameron, Glasgow.

1824.

TO JAMES BLUNDELL. M. D.
LECTURER
ON
PHYSIOLOGY AND MIDWIFERY
AT
GUY'S HOSPITAL.

SIR,

This small work originally appeared under your auspices, I feel ambitious again to present it to the medical world under the same patronage.

It is gratifying to my feelings that an opportunity is again afforded me of expressing the high opinion I have long entertained of your public and private character.

That you may long continue to enjoy increasing degrees of professional celebrity, as the result of unwearied assiduity and acknowledged skill,

Is the wish of, SIR,
Your obliged and obedient servant,
THE AUTHOR.

LONDON,
Nov. 21, 1823.

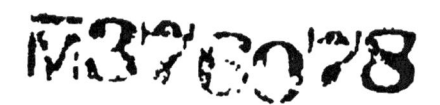

Plummer and Brewis, Printers, Love Lane,
Eastcheap.

PREFACE
TO THE FOURTH EDITION.

THE very favorable reception which [this] small work has met with in the [Me]dical World, induces the author to [sub]mit it again to the press. It cannot [but] be a sense of satisfaction to have [hea]rd, that an attentive perusal of this [sim]ple production has been of essential [ser]vice to gentlemen who have passed [an] examination at Apothecaries' Hall. [F]ew alterations are made in the pre[sen]t edition, thereby rendering it as [com]plete as possible, consistent with the [nat]ure and original design of the work. [S]hould the author receive further [test]imonies of the utility of his little

work, he may be stimulated, at s
future period, to pursue the subject
a more extended scale, introducing
new discoveries which may be m
in this important branch of med
science.

Nov. 20, 1823.

INTRODUCTION.

SEVERAL reasons have induced the author of the following pages to trespass on the attention of the public; more particularly, however, the importance of the subject under consideration, and the repeated and pressing solicitations of friends. These apologies would suffice, if a small work on the subject of poisons were already in print; but there being none expressly confined to this subject, in a concise form, was a further strong inducement for this undertaking. Conciseness, as far as the nature of the subject would allow, without perplexity, has been particularly studied. In addition to the r[e]marks on poisons, the author has su[b]joined a few observations on the mea[ns] to be had recourse to in cases of su[s]pended animation, knowing this to [be] an accident of not unfrequent occu[r]rence, and one requiring immedia[te] assistance. He is now willing to off[er] it to the inspection of the public; an[d] if it should be the means of saving on[e] of his fellow creatures from an untime[ly] end, his trouble will be fully recom[pensed.]

ON POISONS.

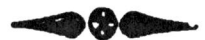

Different plans have been adopted by authors in the arrangement of Poisons, each following some system peculiar to himself; that pursued by Orfila is perhaps the most scientific; but we shall, in this little work, deviate from his system, and class them according to the three kingdoms:—Mineral, Vegetable, and Animal.

MINERAL POISONS.

CORROSIVE METALLIC SALTS.

The symptoms which follow an overdose of the more corrosive metals, are very similar in the different metallic salts. The urgency of the symptoms will necessarily depend on the quantity taken—the form, whether solid or fluid—the state of the stomach at the time, and other occasional circumstances. We shall relate the general operations of this class of poisons, and then the particular ones, and their peculiarities.

When a person has taken a sufficient quantity of any substance to produce deleterious effects upon the constitution, it is said to be an over-dose, or in other words to act as a poison.

General Symptoms.

If Arsenic or Corrosive Sublimate be swallowed, it occasions sickness and uneasiness about the stomach, violent retchings, sense of heat about the mouth and fauces, with a disagreeable taste; the pain in the stomach then becomes very distressing, and blood is sometimes ejected; the bowels are soon affected, and a discharge of offensive matter takes place, frequently mixed with blood, and accompanied with considerable griping and tenesmus. The countenance becomes anxious; the breathing difficult; thirst excessive; skin hot; and pain at the stomach and bowels much increased, particularly upon pressure: then occur cold sweats alternating with flushes of heat, coldness of the extremities, faintness, convulsions, and the most distressing symptoms; which are soon followed by death, relieving the patient from an exquisite state of misery. The pulse is usually small, quick and irregular, but at other times is scarcely disturbed; and is therefore not to be depended on.

ARSENICAL PREPARATIONS.

OXYD of ARSENIC, WHITE ARSENIC, or ARSENIOUS ACID:
(Arsenici Oxydum.)

This mineral, and all the preparations obtained from it, are highly poisonous, even in very small quantities; from which circumstance, it is of the greatest consequence its effects should be watched, when administered for the cure of any disease; and whenever any distressing symptoms make their appearance, it should be immediately discontinued. The same observation will apply to all poisons, particularly the more active minerals; i. e. when any unpleasant symptoms, peculiar to the poison at that time employed, show themselves, it should be suspended for a time, and renewed with great caution.

The Oxyds and Sulphurets of Arsenic, and Arsenites, possess poisonous qualities in different degrees, and will all destroy life if the dose be at all considerable. *Fly water* is commonly a Solution of this mineral.

Symptoms.

For these we will refer the reader to the head of *Corrosive Metallic Salts.* They are generally very distressing, and it is a poison, the operation of which is very energetic in the majority of instances; cases have, however, occurred, where patients have been destroyed without the production of any distressing symptoms, where very large quantities have been taken. One symptom peculiar to this poison is a copious flow of saliva, not having the mercurial fœtor: the evacuations are often green.

Treatment.

Unless our attention is directed to the patient early, there will be little chance of success. As we possess no antidote to this poison, our object is to expel it immediately from the stomach by *emetics*, should it not have excited vomiting, which it scarcely ever fails of doing. *Milk, white of eggs,* and *mucilaginous drinks* should be taken freely, to encourage the vomiting and cleanse out the stomach. *Emollient Clysters* are also to be given, to remove any of the Arsenic which may have escaped into the intestines. It is useless losing time in administering chemical salts, under the idea of neutralizing the effects of the poisons; we have no substance possessed of that power. Sulphurets of Potass and Soda, Lime Water, and Alkalies, have all been used without success. Inflammatory symptoms must be combated by the usual antiphlogistic means.

The *external application* of Arsenic may give rise to all the above symptoms and destroy life.

Tests.

1. A solution of Arsenic is changed yellow by the addition of water saturated with sulphureted Hydrogen.

2. With Sulphate of Copper and Caustic Potass or Ammonia it forms a beautiful green precipitate of *Arsenite of Copper*.

3. By adding to it a small quantity of Liquor Ammoniæ and a Solution of Nitrate of Silver, you will produce a beautiful yellow precipitate of *Arsenite of Silver*.

4. The above results will not, however, enable you to speak decisively as

to the presence of this mineral. It is necessary to reduce some to its metallic state, before we have clear evidence of its existence in a fluid. If any should be rejected solid from the stomach, mix it with some Potass and Charcoal, then submit the mixture to the heat of a candle or spirit lamp, in a glass tube, and the Metallic Arsenic will be sublimed, which possesses a strong smell of garlic, and is very characteristic, this metal only having that odour; it condenses itself on the upper part of the tube, in cubic crystals. This is a property possessed by no other metal. If there should not be any powder in the matter vomited, or in the contents of the stomach (supposing the patient dead), the precipitate obtained in Test 2, or 3, may be submitted to the same process, and a similar result will follow.

MERCURIAL PREPARATIONS.

CORROSIVE SUBLIMATE:
(Hydrargyri Oxymurias.)

Symptoms.

IN adittion to the general symptoms enumerated above, we may notice that the pain of the stomach and abdomen, is generally violent in the extreme; the bowels are speedily deranged, and the evacuations bloody: salivation with the peculiar mercurial foetor, is another well-marked symptom, and one early in its appearance; for it may be remarked here, that none of the preparations of Mercury affect the salivary glands in so short a time as this.

Treatment.

White of eggs and milk, immediately;

the former decomposes Corrosive Sublimate, and throws down an insoluble salt, comparatively mild in its operation. Barley water and linseed tea, or any other mucilaginous fluid, to be taken freely to wash out the stomach effectually. The bowels are next to be attended to; give saline purgatives by the mouth, with emollient clysters. The inflammation must not be overlooked, but treated by leeches, blisters, &c.; and, when the patient rallies somewhat, by venesection. General bleeding will not be proper on the appearance of the inflammation in all cases.

Tests.

1. With Corrosive Sublimate, Albumen forms a white precipitate of *Submuriate of Mercury;* this test will detect very minute quantities of the Salt.

2. Alkalies form with it a red or yellowish precipitate.

3. Liquor Ammoniæ gives a white precipitate.

4. Reduction of the metal with flux (Potass. and Charcoal), is the only decisive test.

Some other preparations of Mercury act in a similar manner, but with much less violence; such as the Red Oxyd, Nitrates, Sulphurets, &c. The plan of treatment would be similar, and the tests the reduction of the metal.

ANTIMONIAL PREPARATIONS.

EMETIC TARTAR:
(*Antimonium Tartarizatum.*)

Symptoms.

THE vomiting, which is the first symptom, is very distressing and urgent; it is soon followed by pain in the stomach; spasm of the oesophagus; great prostration of strength; a quick small pulse: colicky pains soon attack the bowels, and violent purging succeeds; breathing, anxious and hurried; cold perspirations and other symptoms as above.

Treatment.

Decoction of Oak Bark, Infusion of Galls, Sulphuret of Potass, and common Tea, all decompose the Tartar Emetic; and should be taken freely, that it may be thoroughly expelled from the stomach; mucilaginous drink and milk are also proper. If the stomach should continue very irritable, give Opiates.—Treat other symptoms according to their nature.

Tests.

1. With Sulphuric Acid, Lime Wa

er, and the Alkalies, it forms a white precipitate.

2. A Decoction of Oak Bark or Galls, throws down a yellowish precipitate.

BUTTER OF ANTIMONY:
(*Antimonii Murias.*)

Symptoms.

This acts as a powerful escharotic, and when swallowed causes great destruction, giving rise to symptoms of a very distressing nature, as violent as are observed after the Corrosive Sublimate has been taken.

Treatment.

Same as for Tartar Emetic.

Tests.

1. The revival of the metal by flux.
2. It forms a white flaky precipitate with water.

The *Antimonial Wine*, which is often administered by nurses to children, has not unfrequently proved a destructive poison, killing them insidiously; the Sulphurets, and all Antimonial Preparations, act in a similar manner, and the symptoms they occasion must be treated as for the Tartar Emetic.

PREPARATIONS OF COPPER.

VERDIGRIS: (Subacetas Cupri.)

THE preparations of copper are seldom taken or given intentionally as poisons; but from neglect and want of cleanliness, in leaving acid and vegetable substances in copper vessels, these sometimes become corroded, and the Oxyd or Carbonate of Copper is mixed with the food.

Symptoms.

The Salts of Copper give rise to colicky pain in the stomach and bowels: nausea; coppery taste; vomiting of greenish matter, and violent head-ache; severe griping pain in the bowels, with purging often of blood; these symptoms are sometimes succeeded by cold perspirations, convulsions, and death.

Treatment.

Milk, white of eggs, sugared water, and *mucilaginous fluids* freely. If the spasms of the alimentary canal be severe, Opiates will be useful; Emollient Clysters to evacuate and lubricate the bowels.

The Sulphate, Nitrate, Muriate, Carbonate and Oxyds of Copper, and Wines, in which either of these preparations may be present, act in a similar way and require the same treatment.

Tests.

1. All the Salts of Copper are of a green or blue colour.

2. Liq. Ammoniæ, when added to them, forms a greenish precipitate; but if added in excess, the precipitate becomes dissolved, and a beautiful blue solution of the *Ammoniaret of Copper* is the result. If the salt be so much diluted as not to colour the water, this test will detect it.

3. Prussiate of Potass forms a brown precipitate.

PREPARATIONS OF TIN.

MURIATE OF TIN:
(Stanni Murias.)

Symptoms.

Violent vomiting and purgiug, with

spasmodic affections of the stomach and bowels; cramps; sharp quick pulse; sometimes paralysis; with convulsions, and death. It has been mistaken for Epsom Salts, and caused death.

Treatment.

Emetic, if necessary; afterwards milk and mucilagineus fluids; Emollient and Oily Clysters. Opiates to allay spasm of the bowels, &c.: antiphlogistic treatment if required.

Tests.

1. With Nitro-Muriate of Gold, it forms a brownish red, or purplish precipitate, (the *Powder of Cassius.*)
2. With Prussiate of Potass, a white precipitate.

All the preparations of Tin resemble this in their effects, &c.

PREPARATIONS OF ZINC.

WHITE VITRIOL: (Zinci Sulphas.)

Symptoms.

It is generally rejected, immediately that it reaches the stomach, hence it rarely destroys life. It produces a peculiar astringent metallic taste, with a sense of suffocation; but vomiting soon relieves these symptoms; otherwise the countenance becomes pallid and sunk; pulse quick and irregular; bowels always more or less affected: sometimes symptoms occur resembling the Lead Colic, which are succeeded by obstinate diarrhœa.

Treatment.

Alkalies, Magnesia, or Chalk, are the best remedies: After this diluents and

ysters, with Opium if much spasmodic
olic.

Tests.

1. Forms with Alkalies a white pre-
pitate, which is readily dissolved by
ulphuric Acid.
2. With Prussiate of Potass, a blue
ecipitate.
3. With Chromate of Potass, an
ange yellow precipitate.

REPARATIONS OF SILVER.

UNAR CAUSTIC: (Argenti Nitras.)

Symptoms.

It is one of the most corrosive poi-
ns; as we might expect from the re-
lt of its external application. It is,

fortunately, rarely taken as a poison. Its action is similar to the *Corrosive Sublimate.*

Treatment.

The best antidote is mucilaginous fluids, in which Common Salt has been dissolved; this forms a Muriate of Silver, insoluble and harmless: in other respects treat it as for *Corrosive Sublimate.*

Tests.

1. With Alkalies, it forms a white precipitate.

2. With Muriatic Acid, and Saline Muriates, a white precipitate, which soon changes to a blackish colour, by exposure to the air; it may be dissolved by Ammonia.

GENERAL MORBID APPEARANCES.

When life is destroyed by the metalic salts above enumerated, dissection proves that the appearances are similar in the majority of cases. Where *Arsenic* has killed, the stomach and intestines are highly inflamed, often with gangrenous spots in different parts of the former viscus; the villous coat sometimes becomes eroded, and so tender as to be readily peeled off; the peritoneum, throughout the abdomen, is frequently in a state of inflammation. If death has resulted from *Corrosive Sublimate*, the inflammation of the villous and peritoneal coats of the stomach and intestines is more general, and the intestines are sometimes ulcerated. In death from *Tartar Emetic* the morbid appearances are not generally sufficient to account for it. In the other Salts which have caused death, the appearances have resembled those from *Corrosive Sublimate*, but there are no diagnostic marks by which we can tell what poison has destroyed our patient: it may therefore be sufficient to say, that all the Metallic Salts mentioned above, produce more or less inflammation of the stomach and intestines, and of the other abdominal viscera.

PREPARATIONS OF LEAD.

SUGAR OF LEAD:
(*Plumbi Superacetas.*)

Symptoms.

This metal produces effects upon the constitution in a great measure peculiar to itself, giving rise to a considerable derangement in the nervous system; as is frequently observed in plumbers and painters. In a large dose it occa ions pain at the stomach; an astringent metallic taste; sometimes vomiting; obstinate constipation; colicky pains in the bowels; and contractions of the abdominal muscles: these are succeeded by pallid countenance; tremors; sometimes delirium; and if the patient should survive the primary symptoms, paralytic affections seldom fail to make their appearance,

Treatment.

Emetics; Sulphate of Magnesia, dissolved in mucilaginous fluids; Opiates to allay the spasm of the bowels; warm bath; Castor Oil, and purgative clysters, composed of Infusion of Colocynth, or Senna and Salts.

Tests.

1. Sulphuric Acid, and the Alkaline Sulphates form a white insoluble precipitate.

2. Chromate of Potass, throws down a yellow precipitate.

3. Sulphureted Hydrogen, forms at first a brown precipitate, but it soon becomes black.

4. Carbonated Alkalies, form a white precipitate.

Morbid Appearances.

There is merely a stricture about the Colon, or rather a general contraction of that intestine; no marks of inflammation are observed.

The Subacetate, Carbonate, and Oxyds of Lead, and Wines or other fluids, which are either accidentally or purposely impregnated with preparations of Lead, give rise to symptoms similar to those from *Sugar of Lead,* and require the same treatment.

The other Metallic Salts as those of Gold, Platina, Bismuth, Nickel, &c. are never employed as poisons.

CAUSTIC ALKALIES,
AND THEIR SUBCARBONATES.

POTASS, SODA, AND AMMONIA.

Symptoms.

DISTRESSING heat and pain in the fauces, œsophagus, and stomach; nausea; and urinous caustic taste; vomiting, often of blood; intestines soon become affected, and bloody evacuations are the result. *Ammonia* is the most active in its operation, generally causing convulsions and derangement of the intellectual faculties. A large dose of Liquid Ammoniæ has destroyed life in five minutes.

Treatment.

Similar in all cases; neutralize the

Alkali by some mild acid, as vinegar; diluted lemon juice, &c. and give mucilaginous drinks.

Tests.

Alkalies have an urinous taste; they change violets green, and turmeric paper brown; precipitate Metallic Oxyds from their solutions; and form soapy compounds with oily substances.

1. *Ammonia* has a pungent odour.
2. It changes the salts of copper blue.

Potass and Soda may be distinguished by the former becoming precipitated in a state of *Cream of Tartar*, when Tartaric Acid is added in excess; whilst soda forms a very soluble compound with Tartaric Acid in any quantity.

A solution of Platina throws down a yellow precipitate with *Potass* and not with *Soda*.

Morbid Appearances.

Inflammation of the œsophagus, stomach, and bowels, which frequently present a gangrenous and sloughy appearance.

SALTS OF BARYTES.

MURIATE AND NITRATE OF BARYTES.

Symptoms.

VOMITING; purging; violent pain in the stomach and bowels; vertigo; insensibility, paralysis; convulsions; and death. They act with considerable violence and activity.

Treatment.

Sulphate of Soda, of Magnesia, or of Potass, dissolved in some mucilaginous fluid, to be drank freely: they form an insoluble Sulphate, which is inert.

Tests.

The Salts of Barytes form an insoluble compound with Sulphuric Acid and its salts, which will detect very minute quantities of this earth.

Morbid Appearances.

Same as from the Alkalies, and Metallic Salts.

The Carbonate, Acetate, and other soluble Salts of Barytes, act in a similar manner, and require precisely the same treatment.

MINERAL ACIDS.

OIL of VITRIOL: (*Acidum Sulphuricum.*)
AQUA FORTIS: (*Acidum Nitrosum.*)
SPIRITS of SALTS: (*Acidum Muriaticum.*)

Symptoms.

VIOLENT burning pain about the throat, fauces, œsophagus, and whole alimentary canal; fœtid eructations; vomiting of blood; pulse very small and irregular: abdomen tense; great thirst, cold perspirations; convulsions, and death.

Treatment.

In all cases where either of the acids above mentioned have been swallowed, our antidotes must be immediately administered, or they will be useless.

Calcined Magnesia is the best remedy: if not at hand, soap, chalk, or the alkalies diluted.

Tests.

They turn vegetable blues red. Form characteristic neutral Salts with the Alkalies, and effervesce when added to a carbonated alkali or earth.

Sulphuric Acid, forms a white insoluble precipitate, both with the Muriate of Barytes and the Acetate of Lead.

Muriatic Acid, forms an insoluble precipitate with *Nitrate of Silver.* If the fumes arising from it come in contact with Ammoniacal gas, a dense white vapour of *Muriate of Ammonia,* is the result.

Nitric Acid may be known by its red fuming nature; by its forming Nitre when saturated with Potass; and if paper be dipped into the saturated solution, it is converted into touch paper. It forms no precipitate with the salts used to test the other acids.

Morbid Appearances.

If the Acids be concentrated, they occasion complete disorganization and destruction of the parts with which they come in contact: the lining membrane of the æsophagus, stomach, and intestines, is in a high state of inflammation, and often detached; holes are generally formed in the stomach, with gangrenous appearances surrounding them. The *Nitric Acid* proves most destructive; the stomach is converted into a pulpy, soft, blackish, ragged substance, and completely altered in its character; and from the escape of the Acid, the peritoneum becomes inflamed; and where this acid has killed, the parts which it has come in contact with, are yellow.

The *Oxalic, Tartaric, Citric*, and *Fluoric Acids*, when taken in sufficient quantity and undiluted, will give rise to very violent symptoms, and even destroy life; many instances of which have unfortunately happened by the *Oxalic Acid*, or *Acid of Sugar*.

Tests.

Oxalic Acid very much resembles Epsom Salts in its external appearance. It is excessively sour to the taste. It readily detects very minute quantities of the Salts of Lime, forming a white insoluble precipitate with them. The crystals are four-sided prisms.

Tartaric Acid forms a compound of Supertartrate of Potass, when added in excess to a solution of Potass.

Citric Acid crystallizes in rhomboidal prisms, and is the basis of Lemon Juice.

Fluoric Acid has a suffocating smell, and possesses the property of corroding glass, acting upon the silex which it contains.

These, with some other acids which it will be unnecessary to enumerate, produce symptoms, &c., similar to the Mineral Acids, and require a similar mode of treatment. viz. Magnesia, Chalk, Soap, &c.

SALT PETRE: (*Potassæ Nitras.*)

Symptoms.

Violent pain in the stomach, with spasm and a sense of cold; vomiting and purging of blood: very irregular pulse; great prostration of strength; syncope; coldness of the extremities; clammy perspiration; involuntary stools, and speedy dissolution: if the primary symptoms should not destroy, the nervous system becomes more particularly deranged, and paralysis is the consequence.

Treatment.

Emetics, mucilaginous drinks, milk, and emollient purgatives and clysters.

Tests.

1. Crystal six-sided prisms.
2. Detonates on burning coals.
3. When mixed with Sulphuric Acid, red nitrous fumes escape.

Morbid Appearances.

Same as are observed in cases of death from the Corrosive Metals.

PHOSPHORUS.

Symptoms.

Most distressing pain and heat in the

stomach, which are more urgent if the poison be dissolved; besides this, it occasions other symptoms as observed in the Corrosive metals.

Treatment.

It is advisable to expel it from the stomach as speedily as possible; it has been recommended to distend the stomach with food, and then to excite vomiting and give diluents freely. The operation is less violent, the more it is excluded from the air.

Tests.

Its peculiar odour, and general properties, will commonly enable any person to detect it. If dissolved in oil, it is luminous in a dark room.

Morbid Appearances.—See Corrosive Metals.

VEGETABLE POISONS.

NARCOTICS.

OPIUM AND ITS PREPARATIONS.

Symptoms.

This is one of the most common and destructive poisons of this class, and produces symptoms common to all vegetable narcotics. A full dose of *Opium* occasions immediate insensibility; with slow pulse; stertorous breathing; dilated pupil: greatest difficulty in being roused: the countenance is at first flushed, but soon becomes pallid; the pulse then becomes quick and irregular; sometimes convulsions and paralysis precede dissolution. Vomiting is not an usual symptom when the dose is large.

Treatment.

Sulphate of Zinc, gr. viij. vel gr. x. every ten minutes, till vomiting is excited: or Sulphate of Copper, gr. j. to gr. iij.; tickle the throat with a feather, and use every possible means to evacuate the stomach: it will be advisable to pass an elastic tube down the œsophagus and thus introduce emetics, if the patient cannot swallow: the person must be kept in constant motion and exercise by able assistants. In some cases it will be proper to open the jugular vein, to relieve the vessels of the brain from a state of congestion. If scarcely any pulse, Wine, Brandy, and Ammonia, should be introduced into the stomach. Acids should never be given till we are thoroughly convinced no Opium remains in the stomach. Active purgatives both by the mouth and per anum. Coffee may be drank freely. Saline purgatives and effervescing draughts are useful when the patient is recovering. Artificial respiration if required.

Children are often very much injured, and sometimes destroyed, by the too free use of *Syrup of Popies*, it gives rise to drowsiness, insensibility, and convulsions. Treatment here will be Ammonia, Brandy diluted, and Wine with the warm bath.

We are possessed of no tests by which we can distinguish poisons of this class, and can only conjecture they have been taken, by their taste or smell, and the symptoms present.

In general no morbid appearances are evident.

HENBANE *(Hyoscyamus Niger,)* HEMLOCK *(Conium Maculatum,)* STRONG-SCENTED LETTUCE *(Lactuca Virosa,)* WATER HEMLOCK *(Cicuta Virosa,)*

Deadly Night-shade (*Atropa Bella-donna,*) &c. &c.

These, with some others, produce symptoms very similar to Opium, and require the same mode of treatment.

Monkshood (*Aconitum Napelius,*) Poison Nut (*Nux Vomica,*) Spurious Angustura Bark (*Angustura Pseudo Ferruginea,*) Camphor (*Laurus Camphora,*) Poisonous Fungi, with some other, both indigenous and exotic poisons, produce symptoms in some measure resembling those occasioned by the simple Narcotics; they are however more acrid and excite considerable disturbance in the alimentary canal; some exhilarating effects precede their sedative operation, unless the dose be very large; and they more commonly occasion convulsions and spasmodic affections. These have been arranged, by Orfila, under the class Acro-Narcotics,

Treatment.

As for Narcotics, with the free use of diluents. If the breathing be suspended, keep up artificial respiration.

ACRID VEGETABLES.

BLACK AND STINKING HELLEBORE (*Helleborus Niger et Fœtidus*) WHITE HELLEBORE (*Veratrum Album,*) SQUIRTING CUCUMBER (*Momordica Elaterium,*) GAMBOGE (*Stalagmitis Cambogioides,*) EUPHORBIUM, *several species;* SAVINE (*Juniperus Sabida,*) MEADOW SAFFRON (*Colchicum Autumnale,*) SQUILL (*Scilla Maritima,*) several species of RANUNCULUS, &c. &c.

Symptoms.

All these vegetables, in over-doses, and many others, occasion an acrid taste; burning sensation about the mouth and fauces; constriction of the fauces; pain in the stomach and bowels; distressing vomiting and purging, often of blood; succeeded by insensibility, difficulty and shortness of breath and convulsions, and most of them will produce miscarriage.

Treatment.

Mild emetics, mucilaginous diluents, milk, emollient laxatives, and clysters. If the vomiting, after the poison has been thoroughly expelled, should continue to distress the patient, mild opiates are proper.

Morbid Appearances.

Sometimes, in the more acrid vegetables, there is some inflammation of the stomach and bowels; but we cannot generally depend upon these appearances in poisoning from vegetable substances, as they frequently destroy, has an unpleasant smell, and there is often a great aversion to liquids; stomach and bowels are tense and tender, satyriasis, sometimes in a very distressing degree; frequently bloody evacuations; blood is also frequently ejected by vomiting, and passed with the urine; sometimes convulsions and tetanus, and at times abortion.

Treatment.

Diluent emetics; mucilaginous draughts, in which Gum Arabic is dissolved, in abundance; warm bath; clysters of oil. The antiphlogistic treatment is generally required, with opiates.

Morbid Appearances.

Inflammation of the stomach and bowels; also of the kidneys, ureters, and bladder; sometimes the penis is in a gangrenous state.

BITES OF SNAKES, VIPERS, VENOMOUS SERPENTS, &c.

Symptoms.

Acute pain and swelling of the part bitten, which soon extends over the limb; nausea and intoxicating symptoms soon come on, succeeded by delirium; the part bitten becomes livid, and often gangrenous; pulse quick and irregular; breathing difficult and anxious; often bilious vomiting; sometimes impossibility of swallowing, with convulsions.

Treatment.

If possible remove the parts bitten, by excision; then use some caustic application. Oil and Ammonia are generally preferred; in the West Indies they employ Eau de Luce, the action of which depends on the Ammonia it contains. Give Brandy, Ammonia, and other stimulants, with Opiates. Arsenic has been recommended in doses of gr. ss. or gr. j., and it is said, that this practice has been successful. (Vide Medico-Chirurgical Transactions.)

The bites of some venomous insects sometimes occasion unpleasant symptoms; but local applications will generally be sufficient to cure them. If possible, remove the poison; oil applied to the part will often relieve; at other times some evaporating spirituous lotion is necessary, to subdue the inflammation which exists.

MUSCLES, LOBSTERS, CRABS, AND OTHER FISH.

Symptoms.

Uneasiness and pain about the stomach, with sickness and head-ache;

vertigo; redness and swelling of the face; generally a species of nettle-rash all over the body; shortness of breath; rarely, cold extremities, delirium and convulsions.

Treatment.

Emetics, diluents, and purgatives; stimulants and opiates if necessary.

Means to be resorted to in cases where animation is suspended, from drowning, hanging, or breathing deleterious airs.

FROM DROWNING.

First remove all clothes, and then convey the patient to a convenient and airy situation; artificial respiration is now to be commenced, by inflating the lungs from the nose by a pair of bellows passed up one nostril; or with your own mouth, if no other convenience be at hand: when the proper apparatus can be readily procured, that is best for the purpose; after each inflation the lungs must be again emptied, by pressure made on the chest. Wrap the body in warm blankets, and apply warmth to the body in any gradual manner. It is useless and improper to rub the body with any stimulating application. Apply hot water to the feet, or warm bricks. Introduce an elastic tube into the stomach, in order to convey stimulating fluids into that organ, as Brandy, Wine, &c.

The employment of Tobacco clysters is decidedly bad practice.

When respiration becomes natural, we suspend our artificial operations; and as soon as the patient is able to swallow, give wine and water, and nourishing food. Never leave the person until he has perfectly recovered his senses. If Oxygen Gas be at hand, it may be employed. Electricity has been considered by some as an useful adjunct; it may be tried.

FOR HANGING.

A similar plan of treatment is necessary. Bleeding is often required here, from the jugular vein, to relieve the vessels of the brain and lungs; it should only be in a small quantity.

FROM NOXIOUS VAPORS.

Similar treatment necessary. Here the temperature of the body is generally above the natural standard, and cold water should be suddenly dashed over the body, in addition to the other means. It is likewise very desirable, if possible to substitute Oxygen Gas fo the atmospheric air, in these cases.

When suffocation is occasioned by substances lodging in the air passage and thus obstructing respiration, it is often necessary to perform the operation of Bronchotomy: here two methods have been recommended; one dividing the rings of the Trachea longitudinally; the other making an opening between the Thyroid and Cricoid Cartilages: each operation has its advocates, but we should prefer the former.

Papaver Somniferum   Common White Poppy

PAPAVER SOMNIFERUM—PAPAVER ALBUM.

White Poppy.

...psulæ; et capsularum immaturarum ...uccus concretus.

...*ss* **XIII. POLYANDRIA.**—Order I. **MONOGYNIA.**

Natural Order. RHŒADES.

...eric Character. Corolla four-petalled *...alyx* two-leaved. *Capsule* one-celled, opening by pores under the persistent stigma.

...cific Character. Calyces and capsules smooth; leaves incised and embracing the stem.

This species of poppy is a native of

Asia, and is found wild in the south of Europe, where the seeds had probably been accidentally scattered; it is also cultivated in this country, flowering in July.

The root is annual, tapering, and branched. The stalk is erect, three or four feet in height, branched, of a glaucous green color, round and cylindrical. The leaves are large, alternate, lobed, deeply cut into various segments, and embracing the stem. The flowers are large, terminal, and solitary; the calyx consists of two very smooth, ovate, concave segments, which fall when the flower expands; the petals are large, roundish, entire, somewhat undulated, and commonly of a white or purple color: the filaments are numerous, slender, shorter than the corolla, supporting erect, compressed anthers: the germen is roundish, with a many-rayed stigma: the capsule is smooth, large, and filled with a great many small seeds.

From cultivation and difference in soil, several varieties of the *Papaver Somniferum* are met with; the double varieties are not at all inferior to the uncultivated plant.

Every part of the plant has the peculiar odor and taste of opium: but the milky juice, which is the active ingredient, resides chiefly in the capsules. The seeds however, when perfectly ripe, contain scarcely any of the narcotic principle, but are chiefly composed of mucilage, and in their native soil are often used as an article of food; they have a sweetish bland taste, somewhat like almonds.

II. HYOSCYAMUS NIGER.

Common Henbane.

Herba et Semina.

Class V. PENTANDRIA.—*Order* I. MONOGYNIA.

Natural Order. LURIDÆ.

Generic Character. *Corolla* funnel-shaped, obtuse. *Stamina* inclined. *Capsule* covered with a lid, two-celled.

Specific Character. Leaves embracing the stem, sinuate; flowers sessile.

This annual plant is a native of England, and grows by the road-sides and in waste uncultivated places, thriving best in rich soils. It flowers in June and July.

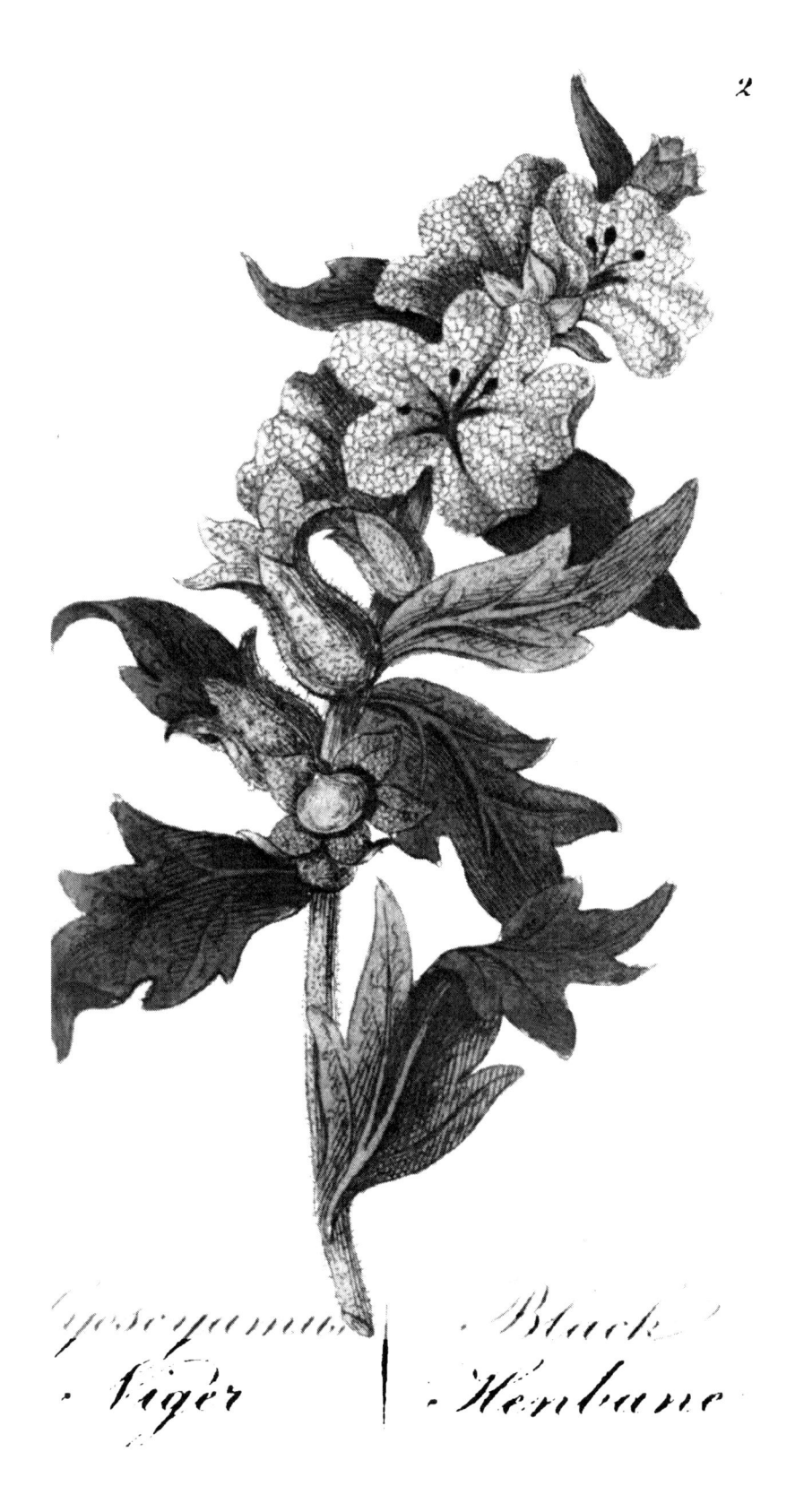

Hyoscyamus Niger | Black Henbane

The root is long, compact, tapering, and fibrous. The stalk is about two feet in height, erect, cylindrical, woody and branched, beset with white hairs. The leaves are large, alternate, embracing the stem; downy, deeply sinuated, undulated, and of a sea-green color. The flowers are simple, placed on terminal leafy spikes; they consist of a short tube with an expanded limb, which is divided into five obtuse segments, of a straw color, and reticulated with purple veins: the calyx is tubular, permanent, and divided into five segments; the filaments are tapering and downy at the base, supporting purple anthers, and are inserted into the tube of the corrolla: the style is longer than the corolla, and ends in a blunt stigma: the capsule is globular, invested with the body of the calyx, and contains numerous irregular brown seeds.

The general appearance of this plant would almost lead us to suspect its deadly nature, and this is confirmed by its strong, disagreeable, and narcotic odor; but it has scarcely any taste, and possesses but a slight degree of acrimony.

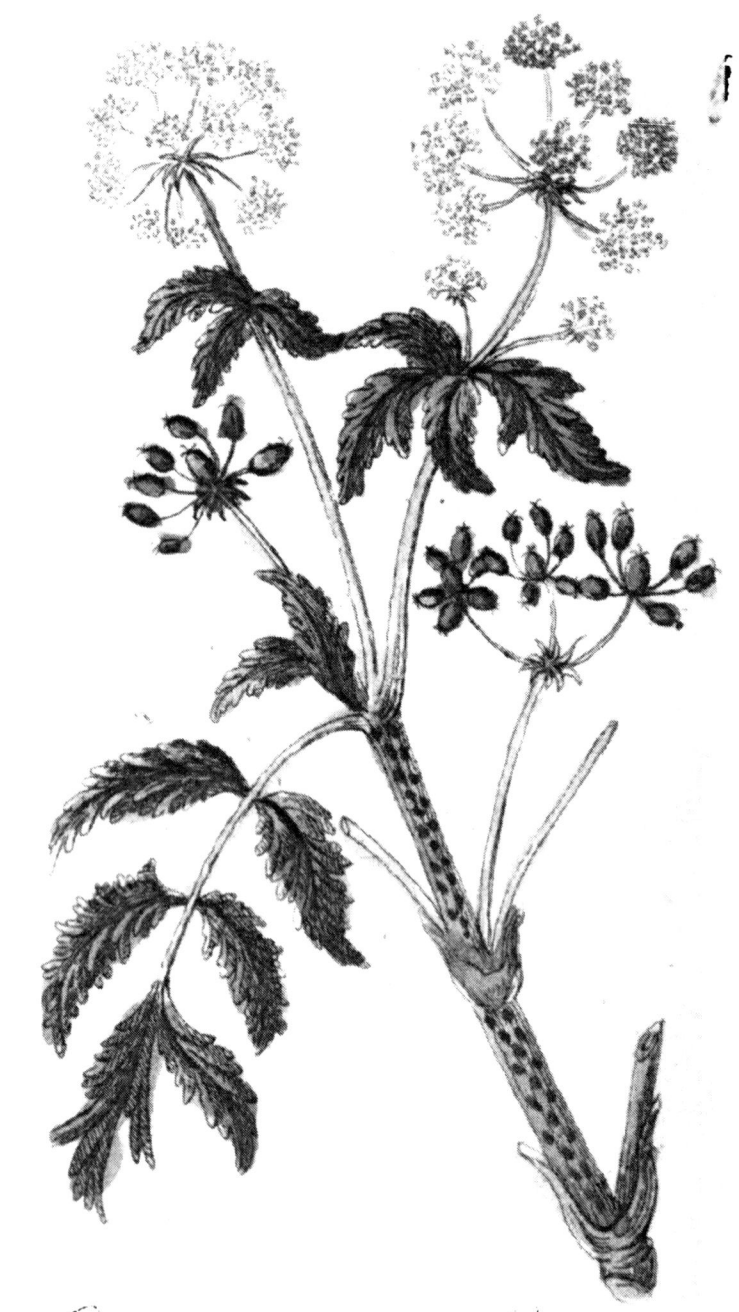

Conium Maculatum | Common Hemlock

III. CONIUM MACULATUM—CICUTA.

Common Hemlock.

Folia.

Class V. PENTANDRIA.—*Order* II. DIGYNIA.

Natural Order. UMBELLATÆ.

Generic Character. **Partial involucrum placed only on one side, three-leaved. Fruit nearly globular, five-streaked, notched on both sides.**

Specific Character. **Seeds striated.**

HEMLOCK is a large blennial umbelliferous plant, growing in the neighbourhood of dunghills, ditches, and in moist shady places, flowering in June and July.

The root is fusiform, about as thick as the finger, yellowish externally and whitish within, exuding when cut, a milky juice. The stalk is cylindrical, from three to five feet high, thick, hollow, branched, leafy, smooth, shining, and beset with purple spots. The lower leaves are large, tripinnated, of a bright green color, standing upon long foot-stalks, which proceed from the joints of the stem; the smaller or upper leaves are bipinnate. The flowers are forming open, numerous, umbels, which are both partial and universal. The involvcrum consists of from three to seven short, reflected, lance-shaped leaflets, white at the margin: the partial involucrum is composed of three or four leaflets, which are disposed on the external side of the umbel. The flowers are small, composed of five petals, unequal, heart shaped, and inclining inwards; with an entire calyx; stamina the length of the petals, supporting whitish anthers; the styles are filiform, larger than the petals, diverging and terminating in round stigmas. The fruit is oval, striated, containing two brownish seeds.

IV. CICUTA VIROSA.

Water Hemlock.

Class V. PENTANDRIA.—*Order* II. DYGINIA.

Natural Order. UMBELLATÆ.

Generic Character. Fruit subovate, sulcated.

Specific Character. Umbel opposite; petioles marginate, obtuse.

ROOT perennial, thick, hollow, and beset with numerous fibres. Stalk thick, round, striated, smooth, and about four feet high. Leaves pinnated: leaflets usually in ternaries, spear-shaped and serrated. Flowers in large expanding umbels. Partial involucrum composed of several short, bristle-

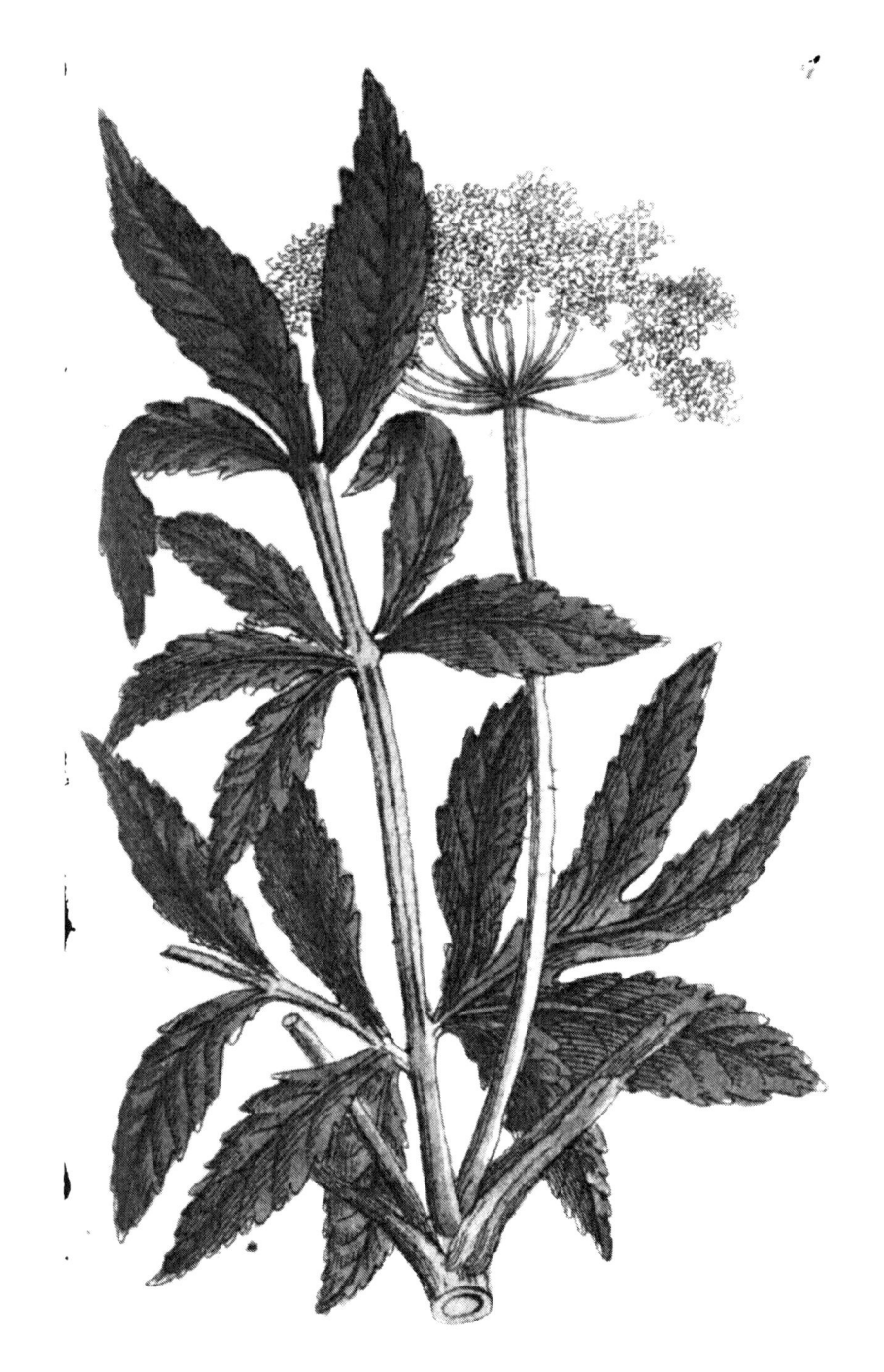

Cicuta Virosa | Water Hemlock

shaped leaves. Calyx scarcely to be seen. Florets uniform, fertile; each consisting of five ovate, greenish white petals: filiments five, longer than the petals: anthers simple and purplish: stigmas simple; fruit egg-shaped.

V. LACTUCA VIROSA.

Strong-scented Lettuce.

Herba.

Class XIX. SYNGENESIA.—*Order* I. ÆQUALIS.

Natural Order. COMPOSITÆ SEMI-FLOSCULOSÆ.

Generic Character. *Receptacle* naked. *Calyx* imbricate, cylindrical, with a membranous margin. *Pappus* simple, stipitate. *Seed* even.

Specific Character. Leaves horizontal; carina pointed and toothed.

THIS plant grows on the banks of ditches, flowering in July and August.

The stalk is about three feet in height, erect, slender, round, prickly

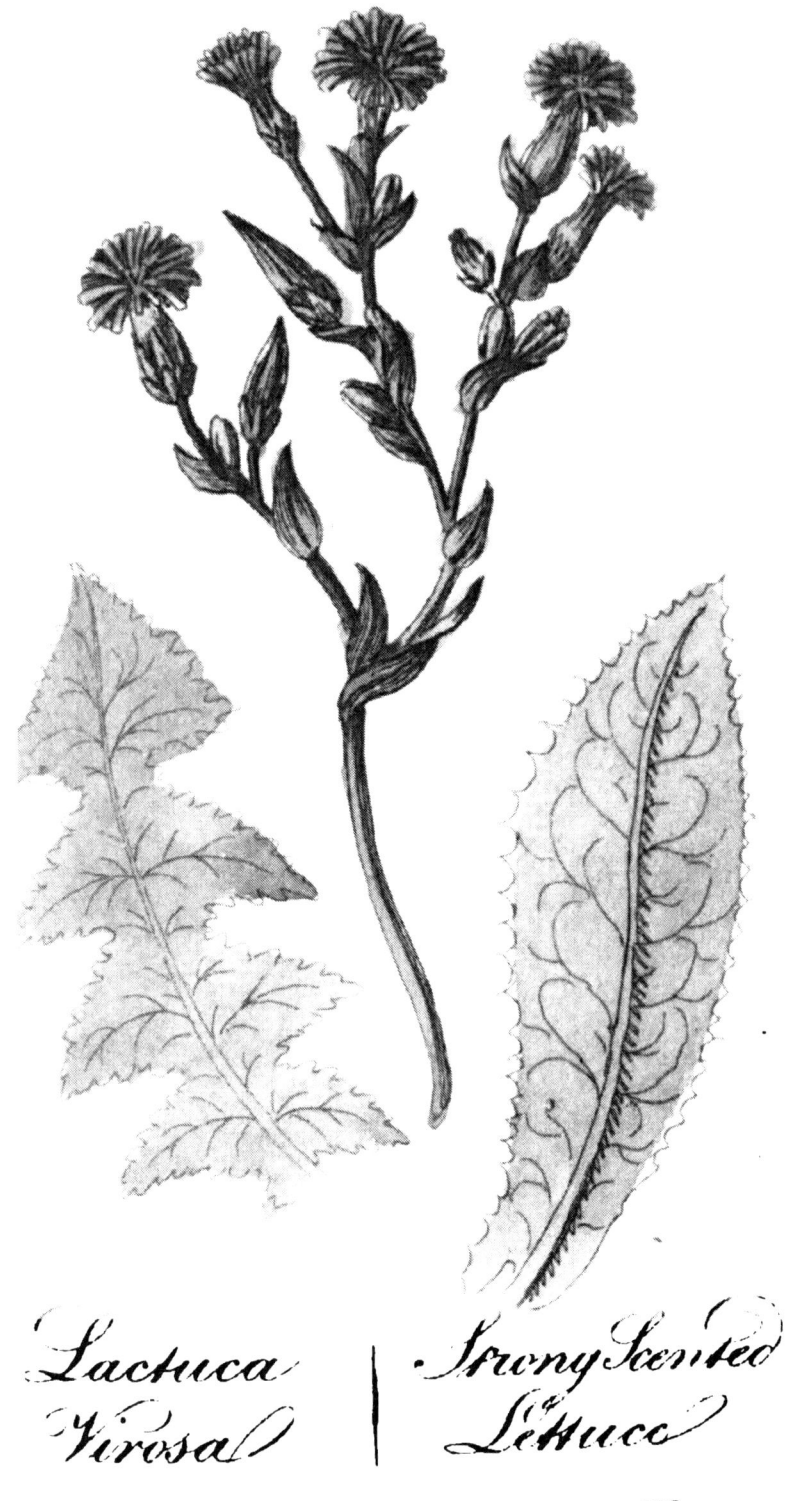

Lactuca Virosa | Strong Scented Lettuce

below, and smooth above. The leaves are smoothish and toothed, the lower ones obovate and undivided; those of the stalk smaller, often lobed, embracing the stem; middle rib having prickles on its under side. Bractes cordate and pointed. Flowers numerous, compound, of a yellow color, furnished with small scaly leaves; calyx oblong, and composed of small lanceolate scales: the corolla consists of florets scarcely longer than the calyx. Seeds elliptical, compressed, black and striated.

VI. ATROPA BELLADONNA.

Deadly Nightshade.

Folia.

Class V. PENTANDRIA.—*Order* I. MONOGYNIA.

Natural Order. LURIDÆ.

Generic Character. Corolla bell-shaped. *Stamina* distant. *Berry* globular, two-celled.

Specific Character. Stalk herbaceous; leaves oval and entire.

THIS perennial plant is common in hot and temperate climates, especially in stony and shady situations. It grows in many parts of England, but is seldom to be met with in the neigh

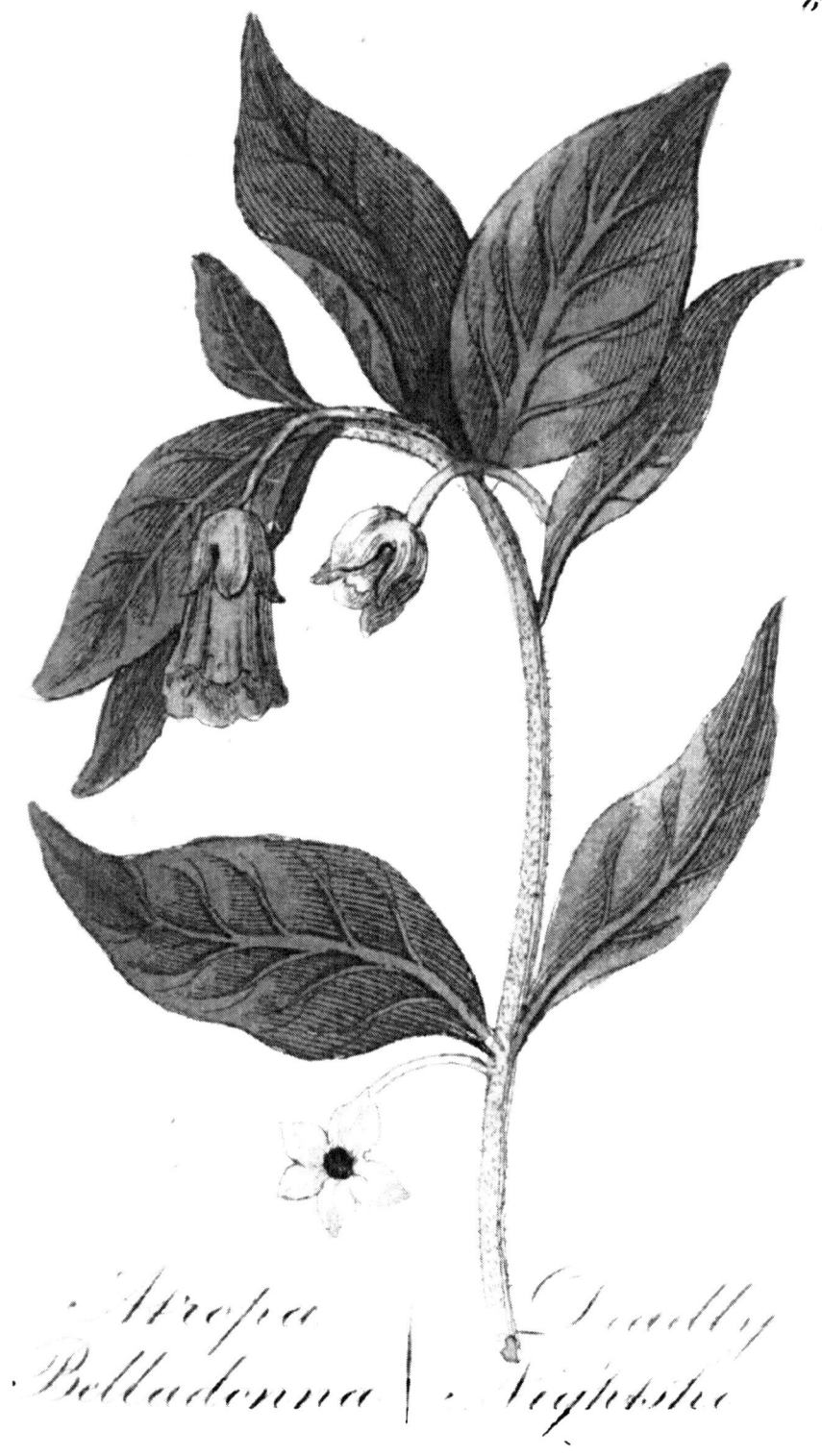

Atropa Belladonna / Deadly Nightshade

bourhood of London. It flowers towards the latter end of June; its fruit ripens in September, and it is frequently cultivated in our gardens.

The root of the Belladonna is thick, long and branched; from which proceed several herbaceous, cylindrical, branched stalks, from three to five feet in height, of a purplish color. The leaves are in pairs, oval, entire, soft, painted, and of different sizes. The flowers are pendant, supported on solitary and axillary preduncles: the calyx is monophillous, deeply divided into five segments: corolla monopetalous, bell-shaped, partially divided into five lobes; it is of a dusky purplish color, and contains five stamens, whose filaments are inserted into the base of the corolla, supporting roundish anthers; a spherodial germen supporting a style wita a divided stigma. The fruit is a roundish berry, contained within the calyx of a blackish color and pulpy, having several kidney-shaped seeds.

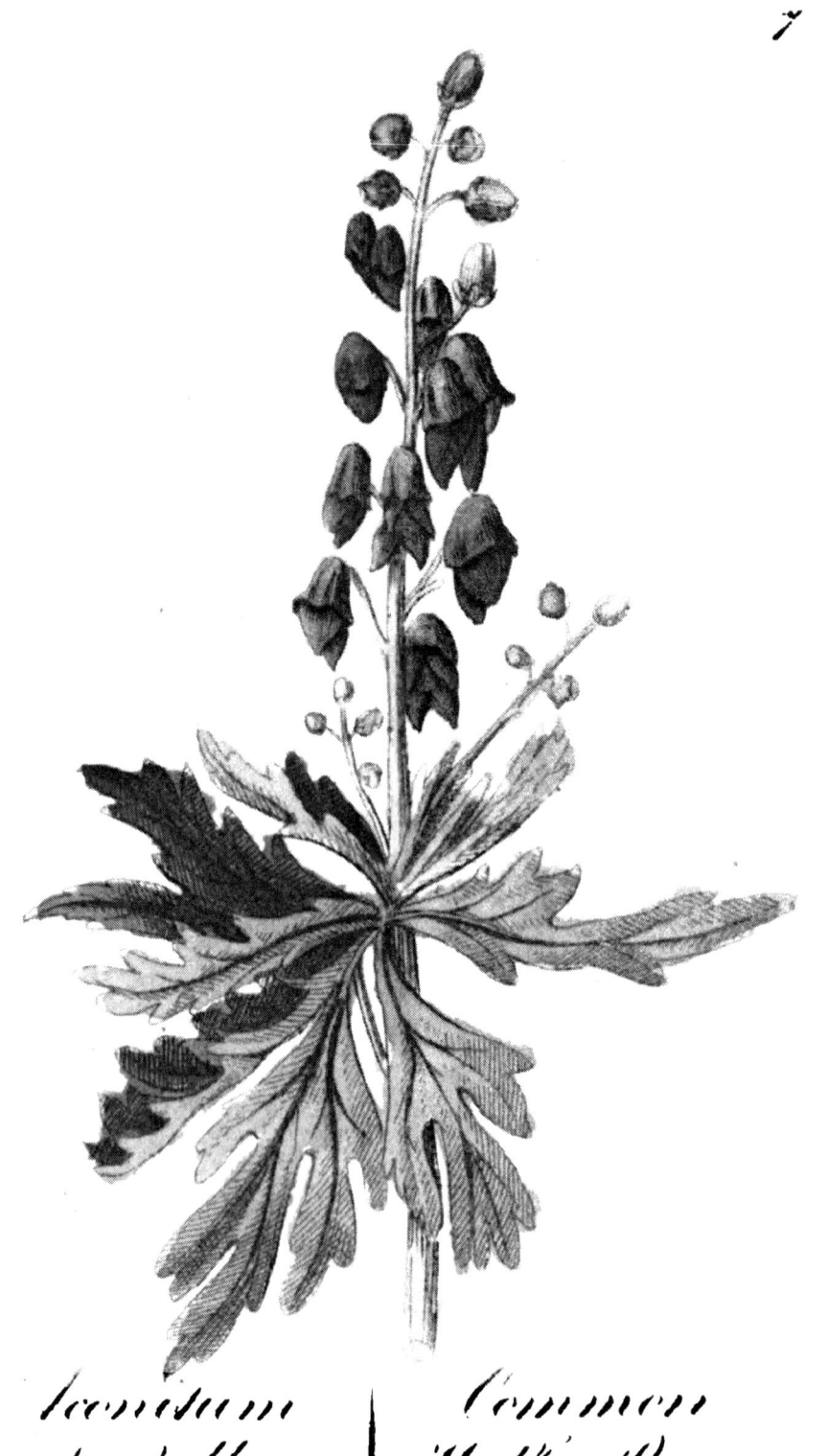

Aconitum Napellus | Common Wolfs-Bane

VII. ACONITUM NAPELLUS.

Wolf's Bane, Monkshood or Aconite.

Class XIII. POLYANDRIA.—*Order* III. TRIGYNIA.

Natural Order. MULTISILIQUÆ.

Generic Character. Calyx wanting. *Petals* five, the uppermost arched. *Nectaries* two, peduncled recurved. *Pods* three or five

Specific Character. Laciniæ of the leaves linear, broadest above, and gashed.

THIS perennial plant is a native of France, Germany, and Switzerland, growing in elevated situations: it is also frequently cultivated as an ornament to our gardens.

The root is fusiform. The stem several feet in height, erect an███ify. The lower leaves are lobed, and deeply cleft, placed on long petioles; the upper ones are nearly sessile, of a dark green color above, and pale beneath. The flowers are placed on unifloral, axillary peduncles, and terminate the stem in a long spike; the petals are of a deep violet color, the uppermost hooded, covering two curious nectaries; the lateral ones roundish, and the lower elliptical: the filaments are spreading, supporting whitish anthers; the germens are from three to five, with simple reflected stigmas.

The whole plant is very deleterious in its recent state; it has a narcotic odour, and a pungent acrid taste: the heat which it occasions in the mouth will continue for some minutes. The acticity of the plant is much diminished by drying, The root is the most active part, but the leaves alone are used medicinally

VIII. DATURA STRAMMONIUM.

Thorn Apple, James-town Weed.

Herba.

Class V. Pentandria.—*Order* I. Monogynia.

Natural Order. Luridæ.

Generic Character. Corolla funnel-shaped, plaited. *Calyx* tubular, angular, deciduous. *Capsule* four-valved.

Specific Character. Pericarps spinous, erect, oval; leaves ovate, glabrous.

The Thorn Apple is an annual plant, and a native of America, but is now found growing in many places in the vicinity of London, and elsewhere

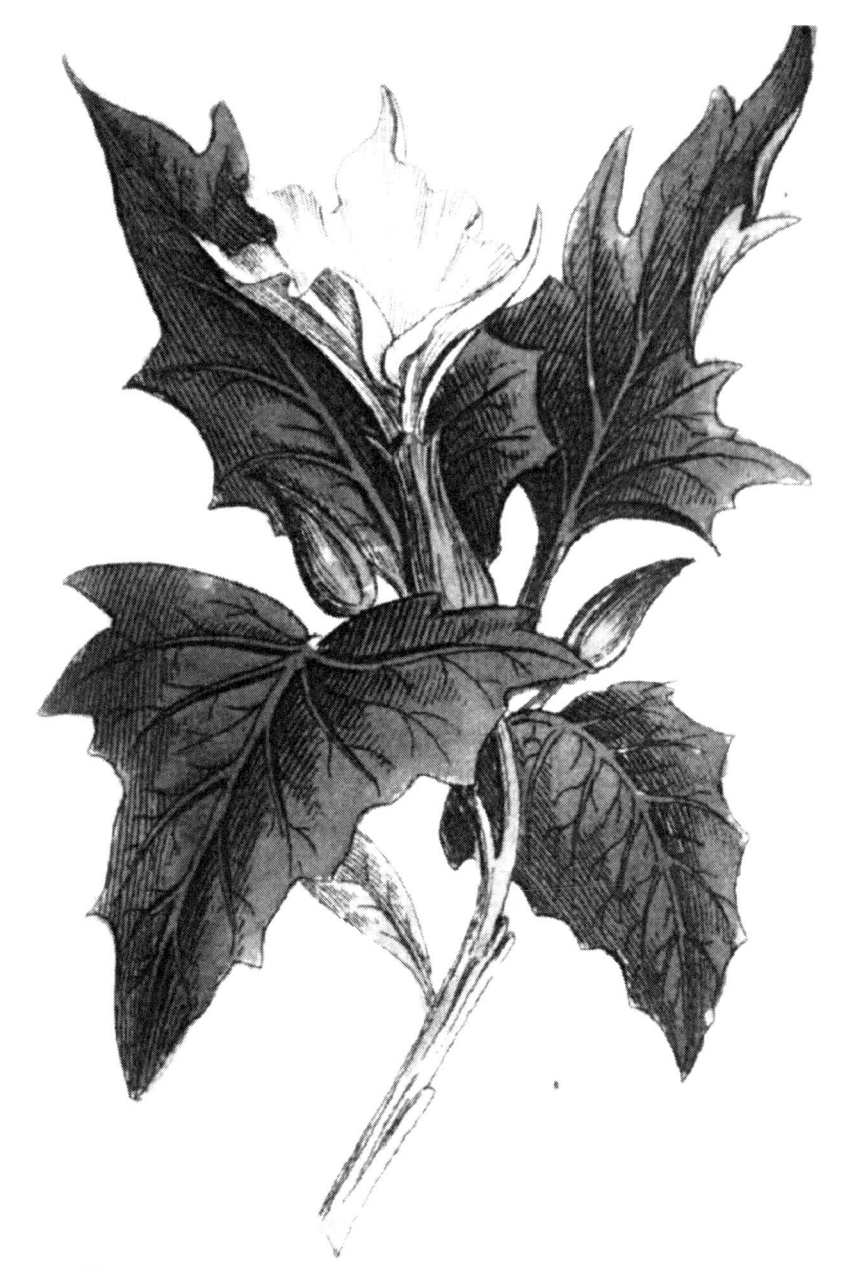

Datura Strammonium | Common Thorn Apple

upon dunghills, and amongst the rubbish thrown from gardens, which generally contains some of its seeds; for it is frequently cultivated, and when it once takes possession of a soil, it is with difficulty extirpated: it flowers in July.

The stalk is thick, round, smooth, spreading, dichotomous above, and rising from two to three feet in height. The leaves are of a dark green color, large, irregularly ovate, pointed at the extremity, angular, deeply indented, and supported by round foot-stalks. The flowers are large, white, axillary, solitary, placed on short erect peduncles: the calyx is one-leafed, tubular, pentangular, and four-toothed: the corolla is funnel-shaped, plaited, furnished with a long cylindrical tube, longer than the calyx. The filaments are slender, adherent to the tube, and support oblong flat anthers; the style is filiform, terminating in a short club-shaped stigma; the germen is oblong, and placed above the insertion of the corolla: the fruit is large, fleshy, ovate, beset with sharp spines, four-celled below, and two-celled above, containing numerous kidney-shaped seeds.

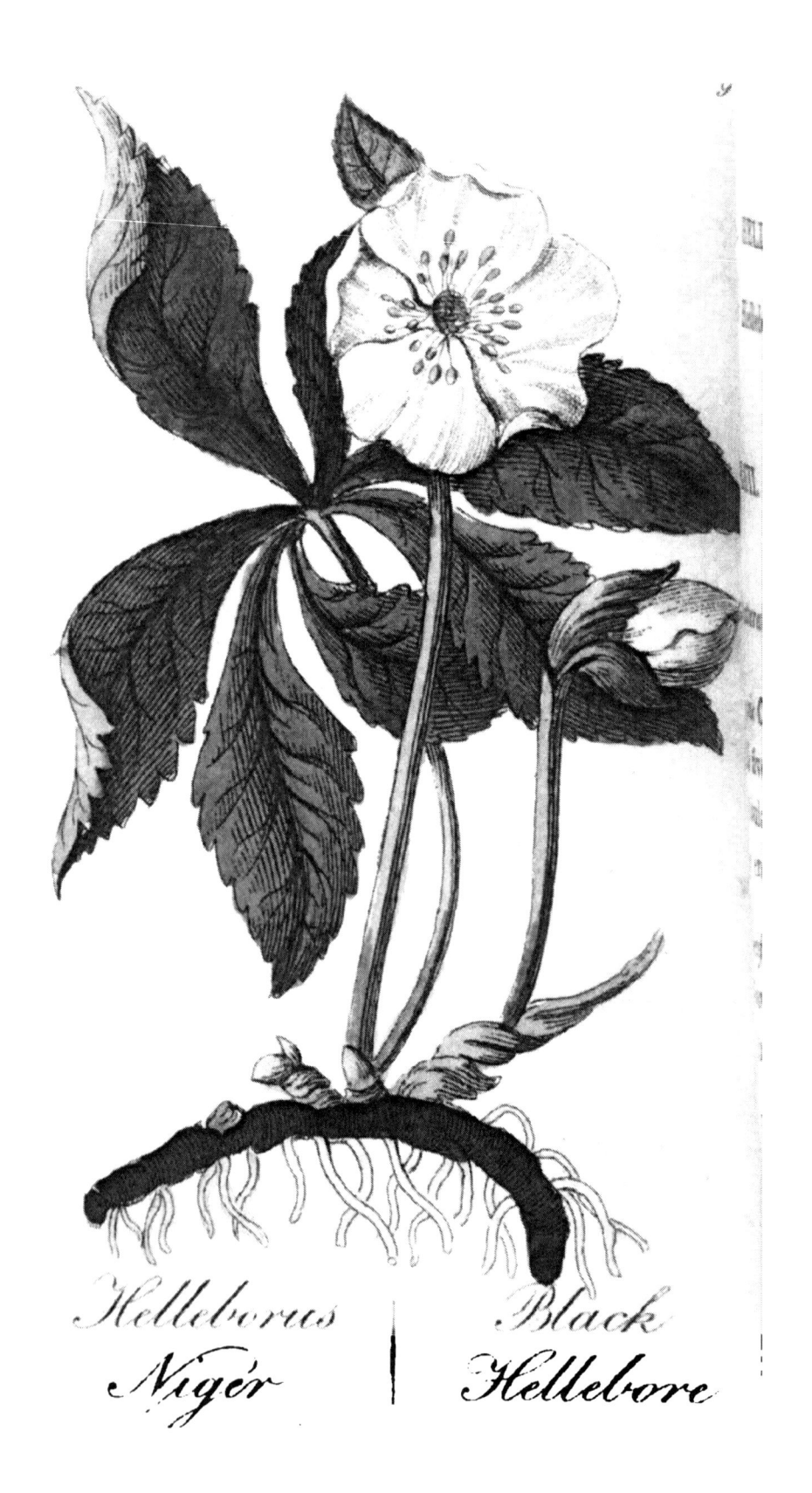

Helleborus Niger | Black Hellebore

IX. HELLEBORUS NIGER.

Black Hellebore or Christmas Rose.

Radix.

Class XIII. POLYANDRIA.—*Order* VI. POLYGYNIA.

Natural Order. MULTISILIQUÆ.

Generic Character. Calyx wanting. *Petals* five, or more. *Nectaries* bilabiate, tubular. *Capsules* many-seeded, nearly erect.

Specific Character. Scape one or two-flowered, nearly naked; leaves pedate.

THIS plant is a native of Austria, the Appennines and Pyrenees, flowering from December to March. It is now cultivated in our gardens.

The root is perennial, transverse, rough, knotted, externally black, and internally whitish, sending off many depending fibres. The scapes, or flower stalks, are erect, round, towards the bottom reddish, and surrounded by an involucre. The leaves are of a deep green color, compound, of a peculiar shape, generally divided into five leaflets, and spring directly from the root, by long footstalks; the leaflets are eliptical, smooth, coriaceous, and the upper half serrated: the floral leaves, which are oval and concave, supply the place of the calyx: the petals are large, roundish, concave and spreading, at first of a white color, with a tint of red, but by age they turn green. The nectaries are eight, tubular, bilabiate, and of a greenish color; filaments numerous, with yellow anthers; the germs vary from four to eight.

Tho roots of several plants have been occasionally mixed with those of the Black Hellebore, and sold as the genuine article; a fraud of the greatest importance to detect, as they possess properties widely different, and some of them are so very active that mischievous consequences have been the result of exhibiting them; for they cannot very readily be distinguished.

The fibrous part of the root, which alone is employed medicinally, is about the thickness of a straw, and six inches in length, of a deep brown color externally, and internally whitish; their taste is bitter and acrid, leaving a sensation of heat upon the tongue; their odor is nauseous and acrid, but much impaired by age.

X. HELLEBORUS FŒTIDUS.

Fœtid Hellebore, or Bear's Foot.

Class XIII. POLYANDRIA.—*Order* VI. POLYGYNIA.

Natural Order. MULTISILIQUÆ.

Generic Character. **Calyx** none. **Petals** five or more. **Nectaries** bilabiate, tubular. **Capsules** many-seeded, nearly erect.

Specific Character.] Stalk many-flowered, leafy; leaves pedate.

This plant grows under hedges and in shady situations, flowering in March and April.

The root is small and bent, with numerous dark colored fibres. The stem is nearly two feet in height, round,

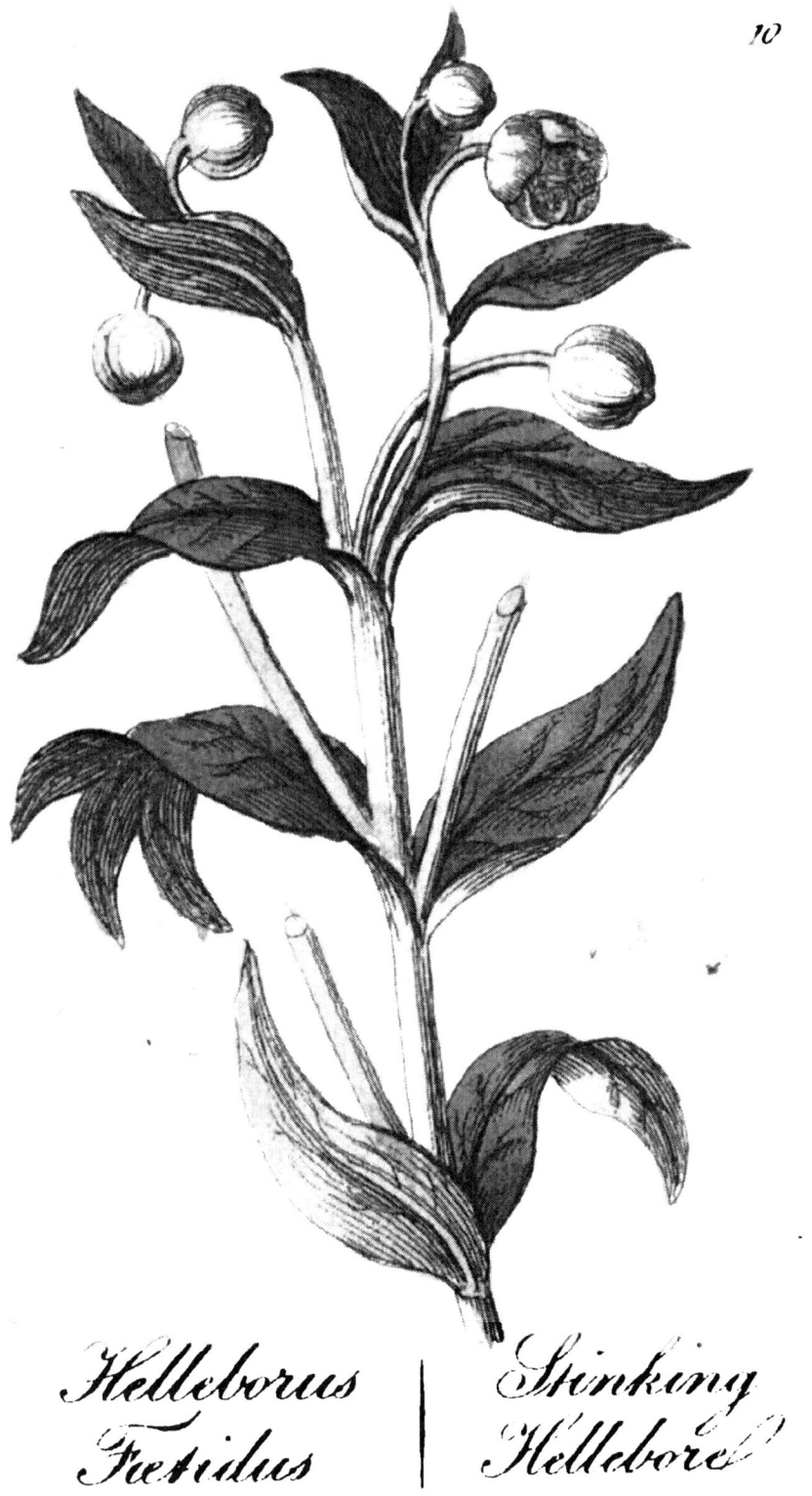

Helleborus Fœtidus | Stinking Hellebore

strong, naked, and towards the top divided and subdivided into branches. The leaves are on long, channelled footstalks, surrounding the middle of the stem, and of a deep lurid green color, and pedate; the leaflets are long, narrow, lanceolate, serrate. At each ramification of the flower stem, are scaly, smooth, alternate, trifid leaves; those near the flowers are oval, entire and pointed. The flowers are numerous, terminal, peduncled and pendent: the petals are five oval, and concave, persistent, of a pale green color, the margins usually tinged with purple: stamina the length of the petals: anthers white: germens three, and resemble those of the Helleborus Niger.

XI. VERATRUM ALBUM.

White Hellebore.

Radix.

Class XXIII. Polygamia.—*Order* I. Monœcia.

Natural Order. Coronariæ.

Generic Character. Hermaphrodite. Calyx wanting. Corolla six-petalled. Stamens six. Pistils three. Capsules three, many-sided.

Male. The same, rudiment of a pistil.

Specific Character. Stalk decomposed above; corollas erect.

The root is perrennial, fleshy, and fusiform, having strong fibres collected into a head. The stem is thick, round,

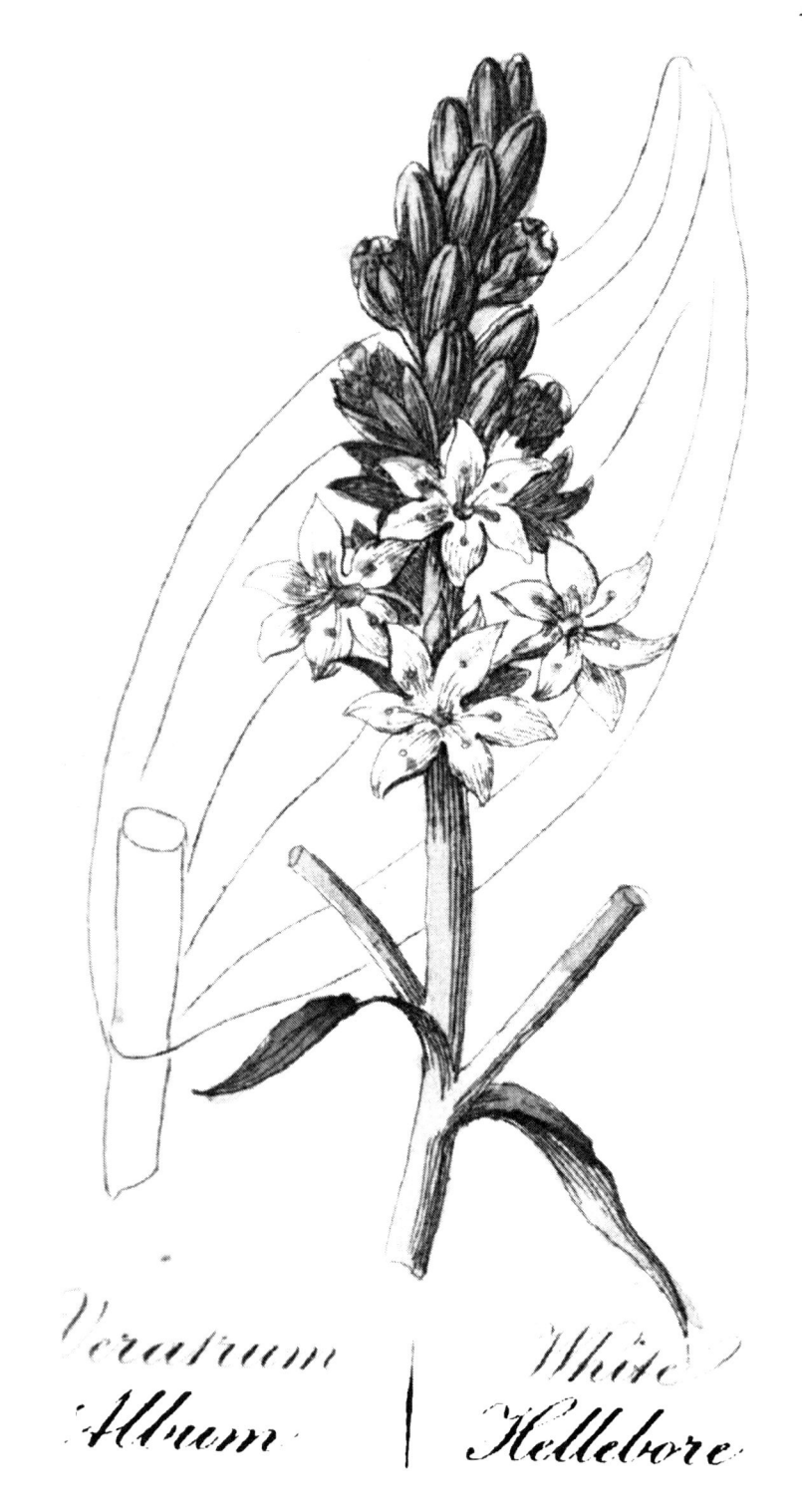

Veratrum Album | White Hellebore

hairy, erect and branching. The leaves are oblong, ovate, plaited longitudinally, of a yellowish green colour, and embracing the stem at the base. The flowers are in long terminal spikes, composed of small alternate spikelets, each accompanied by a lanceolate bracte: each flower consists of six persistent petals of a pale green color: the filaments closely surround the germen, diverge and terminate in yellow quadrangular anthers: the germens are three, in each hermaphrodite flower, oblong, with erect bifid styles, crowned with flat spreading anthers.

XII. COLCHICUM AUTUMNALE.

Common Meadow Saffron.

Radix vel Bulbus Recens.

Class **VI.** Hexandria. — *Order* III. Trigynia.

Natural Order. Spathaceæ.

Generic Character. *Corolla,* six-parted, with a rooted tube. *Capsules,* connected, inflated.

Specific Character. Leaves, flat, lanceolate, erect.

This pe.ennial plant grows in moist meadow-grounds in the more temperate countries of Europe, flowering at the beginning of autumn without leaves,

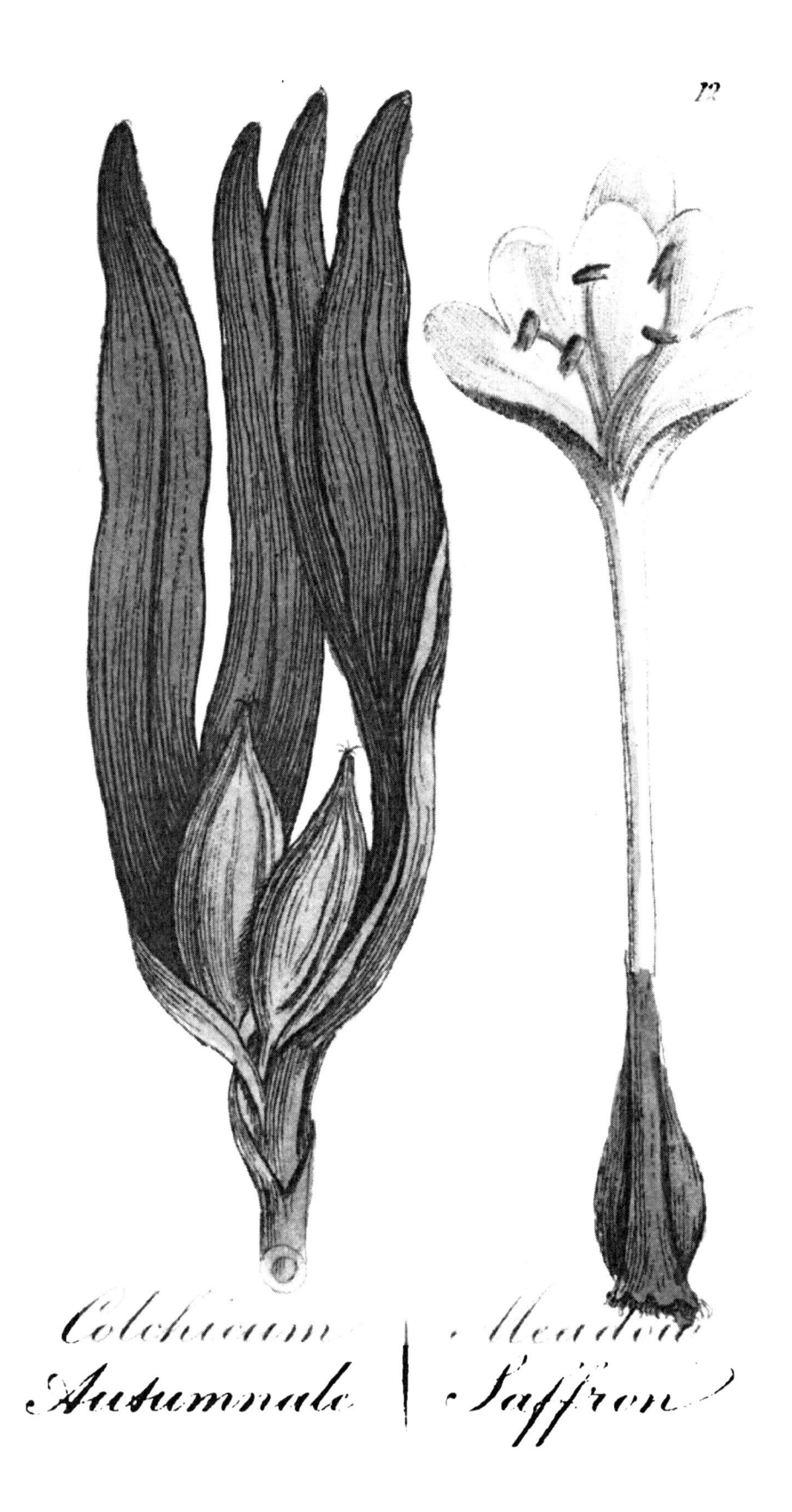

Colchicum Autumnale | Meadow Saffron

and bearing the fruit subsequent to the leaves.

The bulb is double, solid, succulent, and covered with a brown membranous coat. The leaves make their appearance in spring, and are radical, spear-shaped, and somewhat waved. The flowers appear in autumn, immediately succeeding the decay of the leaves; it is large, of a purplish color, and springing from the root by a long naked tube; the calyx wanting: corolla, monopetalous and divided into six lance-shaped, keeled segments, of a pale lilac or purple color: the filaments are tapering, shorter than the corolla, terminating in yellow erect anthers: styles slender and reflexed at the top, supporting simple pointed stigmas: the capsule is three-lobed, three-celled, placed upon a strong peduncle, and containing numerous seeds.

The old bulb begins to decay at the time of flowering (in autumn), at which time the new one is forming, and in the following May is perfected; the old one being entirely wasted, the new bulbs should be dug up at this time, for they possess more activity than those procured in autumn: some, however, recommend that they should be dug up in autumn, but they are certainly much inferior at that time of year; and it is no doubt owing to the bulb being sometimes gathered at different seasons that we have such various accounts of the efficacy of the Colchicum: in autumn it has a sweetish taste, but in summer is highly acrimonious; the nature of the soil is said to have some influence on its activity.

XIII. DIGITALIS PURPUREA.

Purple Foxglove.

Folia.

Class XIV. DIDYNAMIA.—*Order* II. ANGIOSPERMIA.

Natural Order. LURIDÆ.

Generic Character. **Calyx** five-petalled. **Corolla** bell-shaped, five-cleft, bellying. **Capsule** ovate, two-celled.

Specific Character. Segments of the *Calyx* ovate, acute; *Corolla* obtuse, upper lip undivided; leaves downy.

DIGITALIS grows about hedges and and thickets, more particularly in gravelly soils and high dry situations flowering from June to July; it is also cultivated as an ornament to our gardens.

The root is biennial, knotty and fibrous. The stem upright, tapering, roundish, leafy, and about four feet high. Leaves slightly serrated and wrinkled, generally on winged footstalks, alternate, having a dark green upper surface, and the lower one downy: the radical ones are egg-shaped; the upper ones spear-shaped. Flowers numerous and generally grow from one side of the stem; they are pendulous and supported on round footstalks, accompanied by bractes: calyx downy: corolla tubular, somewhat bell-shaped, of a purple color and assuming a mottled appearance within, slightly lobed at the margin; the filaments spring from the tube and support large, two-lobed anthers: germen ovate, supporting a simple style, with its summit cloven.

From inattention to the proper time of gathering the leaves, those of other plants have been mistaken for Foxglove; but such errors may easily be avoided by not collecting the plant till it is in flower, in which state it is most active in its operation. Immediately the leaves are gathered, they must be dried as speedily as possible, and if practicable, this should be effected with the exclusion of light. When perfectly dry they must be preserved in dark situations, free from air and moisture, otherwise they will lose their beautiful green appearance, and become much less active. It is proper to have a fresh supply annually, and we would recommend practitioners, if possible, to superintend the gathering and drying of the leaves themselves.

THE END.

Plummer and Brewis, Printers, Love Lane, Eastcheap.

14 DAY USE
RETURN TO DESK FROM WHICH BORROWED
PUBLIC HEALTH LIBRARY

This book is due on the last date stamped below, or on the date to which renewed.

Renewed books are subject to immediate recall.

~~Aug 28 61~~	
OCT 10 1961	
OCT 4 1961	
OCT 1 1969	
SEP 19 1969	
JAN 20 1971	
JAN 18 1971	
SEPT 22 1976	

CPSIA information can be obtained at www.ICGtesting.com
Printed in the USA
LVOW11s0435290414

383646LV00005B/115/P